Lamine Ghanem Lakhal

Assessment of renal function

Lamine Ghanem Lakhal

Assessment of renal function

ScienciaScripts

Imprint
Any brand names and product names mentioned in this book are subject to trademark, brand or patent protection and are trademarks or registered trademarks of their respective holders. The use of brand names, product names, common names, trade names, product descriptions etc. even without a particular marking in this work is in no way to be construed to mean that such names may be regarded as unrestricted in respect of trademark and brand protection legislation and could thus be used by anyone.

Cover image: www.ingimage.com

This book is a translation from the original published under ISBN 978-620-6-72886-3.

Publisher:
Sciencia Scripts
is a trademark of
Dodo Books Indian Ocean Ltd. and OmniScriptum S.R.L publishing group

120 High Road, East Finchley, London, N2 9ED, United Kingdom
Str. Armeneasca 28/1, office 1, Chisinau MD-2012, Republic of Moldova, Europe
Printed at: see last page
ISBN: 978-3-330-33202-7

LAMINE GHANEM LAKHAL

KIDNEY FUNCTION ASSESSMENT :

Table of contents

1.INTRODUCTION :

Acute renal failure is one of the most frequent organ failures seen in intensive care.

While the incidence of acute renal failure (ARF) after general surgery is around 1%, the incidence of ARF in intensive care patients can be as high as 35% (1, 2).

Acute renal failure is an independent risk factor for mortality (3) (4). Indeed, the development of AKI in intensive care patients has a major impact on short- and long-term morbidity and mortality, and 4 to 5% of these patients require extra-renal purification.

In the medical field, despite advances in diagnostic and therapeutic methods, the assessment of renal function still poses a problem in terms of the ideal marker for early diagnosis and monitoring of acute renal failure.

The simple biological marker creatinineemia has many limitations (dependence on muscle mass, late accumulation in relation to GFR impairment, etc.) (5).

There are other markers used much more to detect the mechanism of renal tissue aggression and not for the diagnosis of renal failure due to cost and lack of clinical studies, the best known of which are (6):

- Cystatin C.
- Kidney Injury molecule-1 (KIM-1).
- Neutrophil gelatinase associated lipocalin (NGAL).
- Interleukin-18 (IL-18).
- β2-microglobulin.

The study of renal perfusion by parenchymal pulsed Doppler, or by semi-quantitative assessment using color Doppler, or by renal contrast ultrasonography, appears to be a promising method for the early diagnosis of renal damage.

Advances in the use of non-invasive techniques (ultrasound) to diagnose and monitor various pathologies in emergency and intensive care settings have made it possible to study renal perfusion using the Doppler method, as part of the assessment of renal function.

The study of renal perfusion by renal parenchymal Doppler probably enables early detection of patients at risk of developing acute renal failure, so that so-called preventive strategies can be planned. (7)

Several methods of assessing renal perfusion can be used in renal ultrasound. They are represented by :

- The semi-quantitative color Doppler renal perfusion assessment scale.
- Contrast-enhanced ultrasound (CEUS).
- renal vascular resistance index (RRI).

Semi-quantitative assessment using color Doppler allows us to determine a scale for evaluating renal perfusion, ranging from 0 (no identifiable vessels) to 3 (visible vessels up to the arterial arteries).

Contrast-enhanced ultrasound (CEUS) measures two indices: mean transit time and relative blood volume. A relationship between these two indices reflects visceral perfusion.

Human data highlight the heterogeneity of the results obtained and the lack of correlation between CEUS-derived indices and renal macro- or microcirculatory data (8).

The study of renal perfusion by pulsed Doppler allows the measurement of two indices:

- Renal resistance index (RRI) deduced from systolic and diastolic velocities

$$Index\ de\ r\acute{e}sistance\ r\acute{e}nal = \frac{Vitesse\ systolique - Vitesse\ diastolique}{Vitesse\ systolique}$$

- The pulsatility index (PI), calculated from systolic, diastolic and mean velocities.

$$Index\ de\ pulsatilit\acute{e} = \frac{Vitesse\ systolique - Vitesse\ diastolique}{Vitesse\ moyenne}$$

As the renal circulation has a non-resistive profile, we use the renal resistance index, as the pulsatility index is used for circulations with a resistive profile (e.g. vessels of both upper and lower limbs).

The renal resistance index has been used as a diagnostic tool and prognostic indicator of acute renal failure in several studies. We find it as :

- Diagnosis of early renal graft rejection (9).
- Method for assessing the impact of ureteral obstruction on renal function (10).
- Technique for assessing the risk of postoperative renal failure (11).
- A prognostic indicator in acute renal failure (persistence or reversibility of AKI) (12).

2. ANATOMICAL-PHYSIOLOGICAL REMINDER :

2.1 Renal structure and function :

The two kidneys are located separately in a cellulo-adipuate lodge in the retroperitoneal space on either side of the vertebral column (13, 14). On average, they measure 12 cm in the long axis and 6 cm in the transverse axis (Fig.1).

The renal parenchyma can be divided into two parts:

- The renal cortex: this is the superficial part of the kidney, containing the renal corpuscles, the glomeruli and the initial and terminal segments of the renal tubules.
- Renal medullary: composed of the renal pyramids (Malpighian). It contains the ascending and descending segments of the renal tubules.

The main renal functions are :

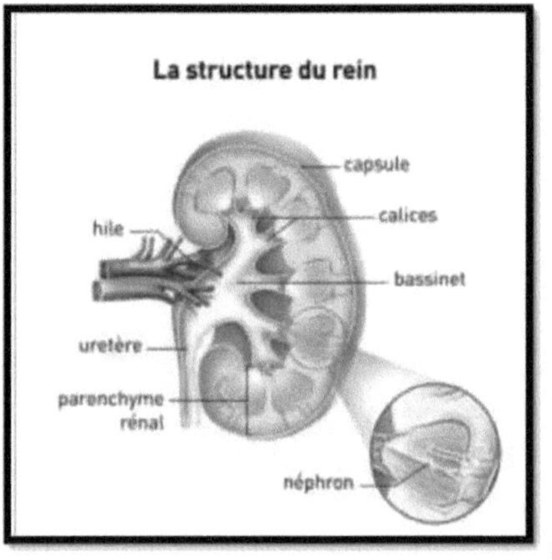

(13)

Figure 1: Anatomical structures of the kidney.

2.1.1 Glomerular filtration :

This is the first stage in the formation of urine. It is a passive process in which fluids and solutes pass through Bowman's capsule. This plasma ultrafiltrate is known as primary urine. In adults, the normal DGF is 120 to 125 ml /min in both kidneys, resulting in the formation of 180 l of ultrafiltrate per day.

2.1.2 Tubular reabsorption function :

Reabsorption is a phenomenon that can be active (energy consumption) or passive, involving any substance essential for maintaining homeostasis and a normal fluid and electrolyte balance (Fig. 2).

The main substances reabsorbed are: water and sodium, glucose and amino acids, urea and the bicarbonate ion HCO3-.

2.1.3 Tubular secretory function :

It requires specific transporters, and this transport is often active (against the concentration gradient), making it possible to increase the excretion of a substance compared with filtration without reabsorption (Fig.2).

Secretion mainly involves metabolic waste (xenobiotics), protons and potassium as part of the regulation of homeostasis.

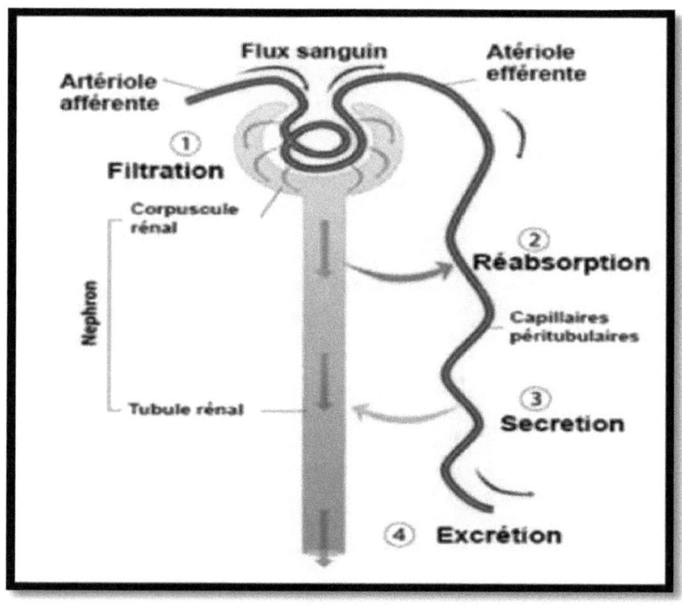

(13)

Figure 2: Urine formation.

2.1.4 Kidney and acid-base balance :

The kidney helps regulate the acid-base balance by eliminating excess acid charges in the form of H+ protons, titratable acidity or NH4+.

It manages the electro-neutral balance by modifying reabsorption and secretion phenomena to achieve a stable Strong Ion Difference (SID).

2.1.5 The endocrine function of the kidney :

The active form of vitamin D [1,25 (OH) 2- vitamin D3 or calcitriol] is produced in the kidneys from its hepatic precursor 25 (OH) vitamin D3 by un alpha-hydroxylase. The activity of this enzyme is enhanced by the parathyroid hormone PTH, which increases digestive and renal calcium absorption.

Erythropoietin (EPO) is produced by interstitial cells to stimulate erythropoiesis in response to changes in arterial O2 partial pressure.

Hypovolemia and falling blood pressure stimulate the renin-angiotensin-aldosterone system (RAAS), which promotes the production of angiotensin II (a powerful vasoconstrictor) and adrenal cortical secretion of aldosterone (sodium retention, secretion of protons H+, and potassium K+).

2.2 **Physiology of the renal circulation** :

The renal circulation (14) has a number of features that determine its functionality (Fig.3).

The renal artery gives rise to arteries called the inter-lobar arteries, then to the arcuate arteries, followed by the inter-lobar arteries.

The inter-lobular arteries give rise to the afferent arterioles of the glomerulus.

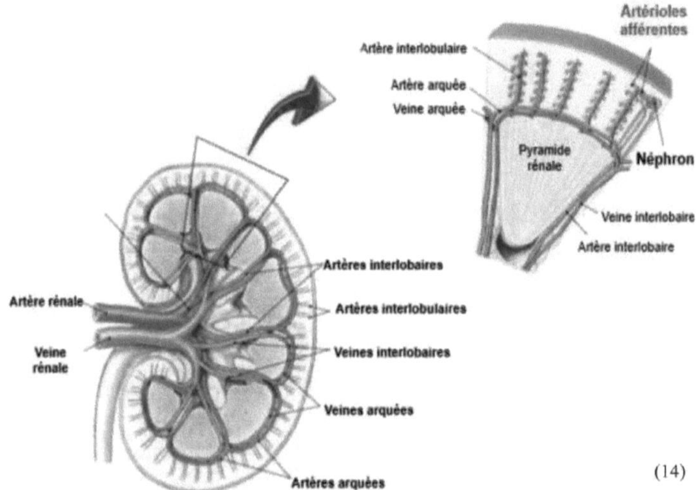

Figure 3: The renal circulation.

Intra-renal circulation comprises two successive capillary networks:

- A glomerular arterioarterial network representing the glomerular microcirculation (Fig.4).

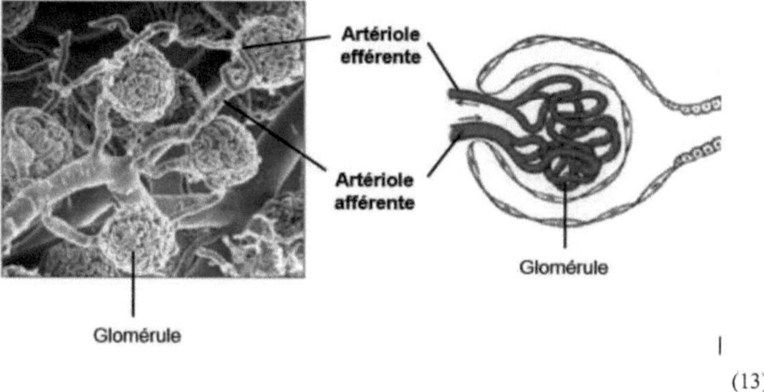

(13)

Figure 4: Circulation of the nephron.

- Another peri-tubular arteriovenous network, representing the postglomerular microcirculation, comprises a dense, abundant cortical segment and a poor, tenuous medullary segment (Fig. 5).

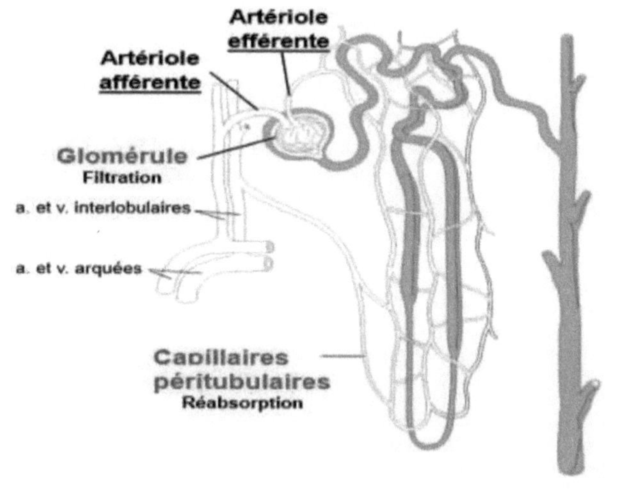

(13)

Figure 5: Capillary beds of the nephron.

Anatomically speaking, we need to focus on a complex renin-secreting formation known as the juxta glomerular apparatus (JGA), formed by direct contact between the glomerular network and a differentiated part of the distal convoluted tubule known as the macula densa (Fig.6).

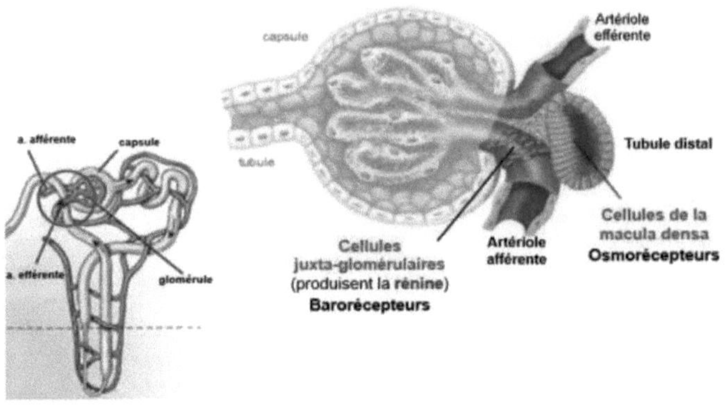

(13)

Figure 6: Juxta-glomerular apparatus.

2.2.2 Glomerular filtration rate :

Glomerular filtration rate (14) depends on the permeability of the glomerular filtration barrier and the difference between hydrostatic and oncotic pressures in the glomerular capillary (Fig.7).

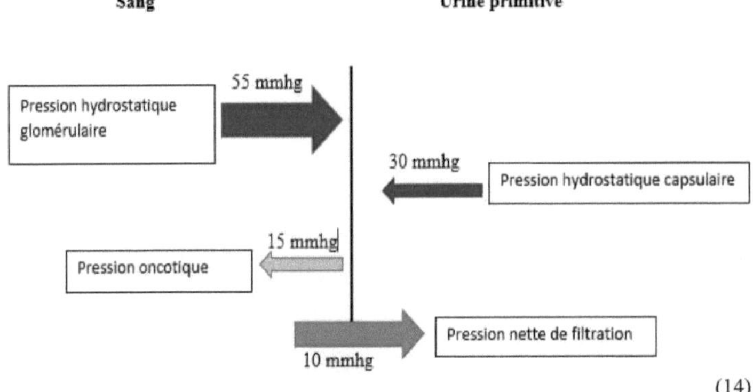

(14)

Figure 7: Glomerular filtration.

Impaired glomerular filtration rate (GFR) defines acute renal failure.

This filtration rate can be deduced from the following formula:

$$DFG=Kf \times delta\ P$$

- Delta P = pressure gradient difference (oncotic and hydrostatic).
- Kf= permeability coefficient of the glomerular membrane.

Glomerular filtration rate represents around 20% of renal plasma flow (RPF), or 120 ml/min in humans.

A decrease in glomerular filtration rate may be observed (14):

- In situations where hydrostatic pressure is reduced (hypotension, shock....).
- Increased tubular pressure (urinary tract obstruction).
- During alterations in the vasomotor balance between the afferent and efferent arterioles.
- In the event of reduced membrane permeability.

Physiological variations in glomerular filtration rate can be seen (15):

- During intense muscular activity.
- In pregnant women, with a 30% increase in GFR.
- Age-dependent: in infants and grandchildren, glomerular filtration rate is low, initially increasing with age, then gradually decreasing by an average of 5% per decade.

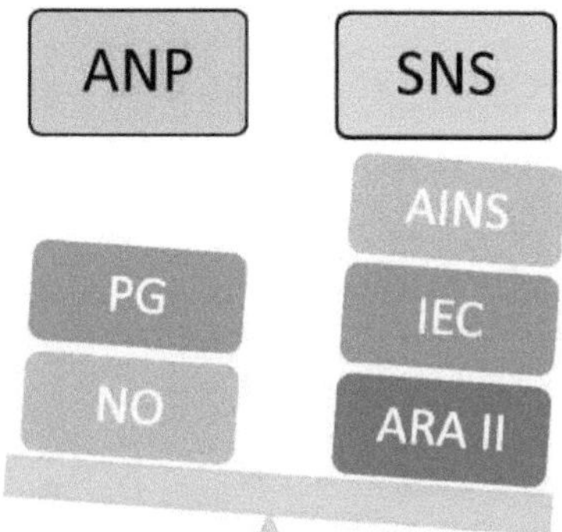

Figure 8: Factors influencing glomerular filtration rate.

NSAID: non-steroidal anti-inflammatory drug; ANG II: angiotensin II; ANP: atrial natriuretic peptide; ARB II: angiotensin II receptor antagonist; GFR: glomerular filtration rate; GTF: tubulo-glomerular feedback; ACEI: ACE inhibitor; NO: nitric oxide; PG: prostaglandins; QC: cardiac output; SNS: sympathetic nervous system.

The regulation of glomerular filtration rate involves a number of other factors, illustrated in figures 8 and 9. Glomerular chamber pressure is the main determinant of GFR. This pressure depends on the interplay of vasodilation and vasoconstriction between the afferent and efferent arterioles. Alteration of the vasoconstrictor tone in the efferent arteriole, caused by anti-angiotensin II receptor blockers (ARB II), lowers glomerular pressure and reduces GFR.

The use of non-steroidal anti-inflammatory drugs (NSAIDs) inhibits the synthesis of certain prostaglandins responsible for vasodilation in the afferent arteriole, resulting in a secondary drop in GFR.

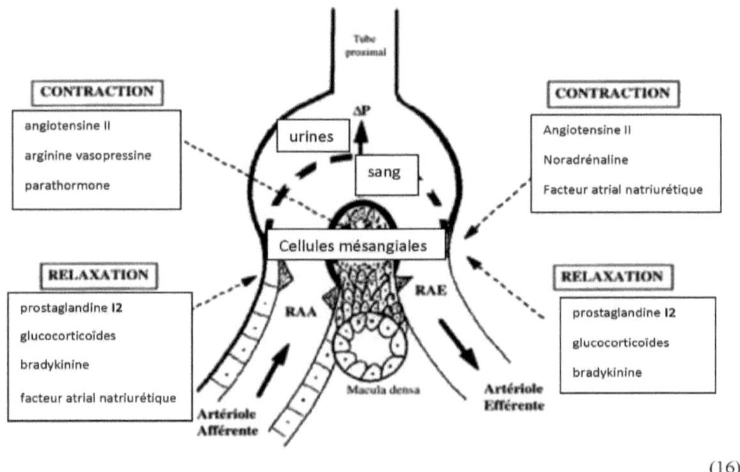

(16)

Figure 9: Regulation of glomerular filtration rate.

2.2.3 Renal vascular pressures :

The main intra-renal vascular resistances are pre- and post-glomerular. Hydrostatic pressure decreases as arteriolar bifurcations take place (14). This pressure is of the order of 55 mmhg in glomerular capillaries, enabling it to remain higher than oncotic pressure and ensure glomerular filtration flow.

Hydrostatic pressure is low in the peri-tubular regions, favoring reabsorption of substances from the tubular lumen into the capillaries (Fig.10).

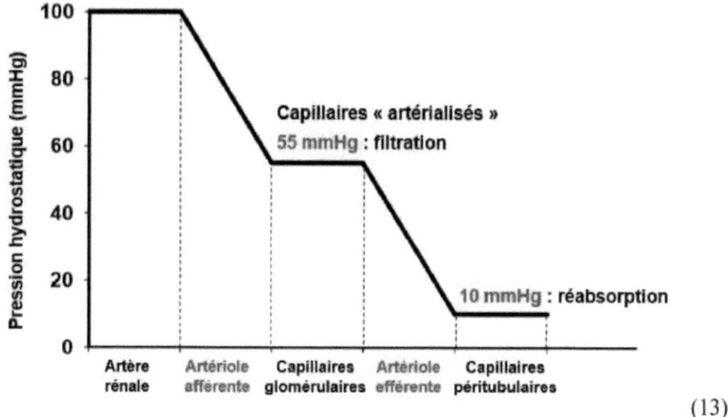

(13)

Figure 10: Renal vascular pressures.

2.2.4 Renal vascular regulation :

There are two types of intra-renal vascular regulation (Fig.11):

- Intrinsic regulation, known as autoregulation, is conditioned by transmural vascular wall pressure (TMWP), which represents the difference between intravascular and extravascular pressure.

Increasing this transmural pressure causes reflex vasoconstriction, and decreasing it causes reflex vasodilation. This is the myogenic theory of peripheral regulation of vascular tone. This regulatory mechanism helps maintain stable renal blood flow between 80 and 160 mmhg mean arterial pressure.

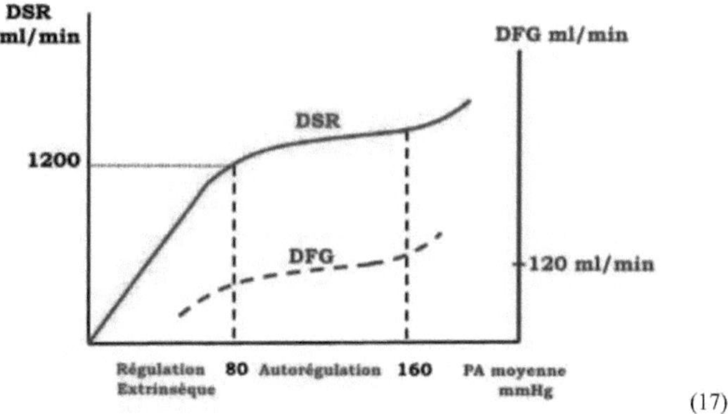

(17)

Figure 11: Regulation of renal circulation.

RFS: renal blood flow GFR: glomerular filtration rate

- Extrinsic, neurohormonal regulation, involving the adrenergic and renin angiotensin aldosterone systems, to manage renal blood flow above or below the limits of myogenic autoregulation.

3. KIDNEY FUNCTION MARKERS :

3.1 Measurement of glomerular filtration rate :

Measurement of glomerular filtration rate is based on the concept of renal clearance:

A substance X eliminated by glomerular free filtration alone (not secreted or reabsorbed by the tubules after ultrafiltration and of low molecular weight).

The flow rate of this substance X (whose plasma concentration is Px) in the glomerular Fultrafiltrat (GFR x Px) is equal to the flow rate of the same substance in the urine (Ux x DU).

The glomerular filtration rate (GFR) can thus be calculated from the blood and urine bioassay of X according to the equation :

$$DFG = Ux \ X \ DU \ / \ Px = \text{Clairance de X.}$$

GFR = glomerular filtration rate (ml/min). UF = urine flow (ml/min).

The ideal substance for reliable measurement of glomerular filtration rate must meet certain conditions:

- Substance completely filtered, not reabsorbed or excreted by the tubular system.
- Substance not metabolized by the body.
- Low-molecular-weight substance, non-ionized and not bound by proteins

The only exogenous substance with the above characteristics is inulin , an extracellular fructose polymer.

Other exogenous substances are now used as filtration markers, such as 125I Iothalamate or 51Cr EDTA, Iohexol (15).

In practice, renal function is often assessed by measuring two biological markers: urea and creatinine.

3.2 Urea dosage :

Urea is a nitrogenous waste product of protein degradation, synthesized by the liver, filtered by the kidneys and eliminated in the urine. Elevated blood urea levels may indicate impaired glomerular filtration rate (18).

Urea accounts for around 90% of total urinary nitrogen in adults. It is produced largely by the liver and to a lesser extent by the kidneys.

The urea level depends not only on renal function, but also on many other parameters, making it a poor biomarker of glomerular filtration. These parameters are represented by :

- Protein intake.
- Protein catabolism in the body.

- The person's state of hydration.
- Gastrointestinal bleeding.

Not to mention the so-called physiological variations:

- Pregnancy reduces its concentration by 30-60%.
- Age: concentration falls in infants (-30%) and rises in adults over 55 (+20%).
- Gender: due to the difference in muscle mass, urea is higher in men than in women (5%).

- Prolonged effort can increase concentration by 20%.
- Prolonged fasting (significantly reduces urea concentration).

3.3 Creatinine levels:

Assessing renal function by measuring glomerular filtration rate alone underestimates tubular function. Glomerular filtration rate can be impaired in all types of renal disease, and is an indirect reflection of non-glomerular pathology (5).

Creatinine, a protein derived from the breakdown of muscle creatine, has the peculiarity of being completely filtered by the renal glomerulus and not reabsorbed by the tubule. It is partially secreted by these tubules, which may overestimate GFR. Its ease of monitoring, both in blood and urine, and low cost, have made it the marker of choice for assessing renal glomerular filtration (5).

The limitations of this endogenous biomarker (creatininemia) are its muscular origin and high volume of distribution.

The main factors influencing its production and therefore its plasma concentration are :

- Age.
- Sex.
- The breed.
- Weight.

The evolution of creatinine levels can be dissociated from that of glomerular filtration rate (19).

Creatinine concentration therefore depends on a balance between muscle production, renal elimination and volume of distribution (which plays a minor role).

An increase in plasma creatinine only appears when glomerular filtration rate falls by almost 50%. A significant rise in serum creatinine is a highly specific but not very sensitive marker of acute renal failure, since a fall in GFR is only detected in 60% of cases by a rise in serum creatinine.

Comparing the increase in plasma creatinine with a baseline value is probably the best way to determine whether renal failure is acute (5).

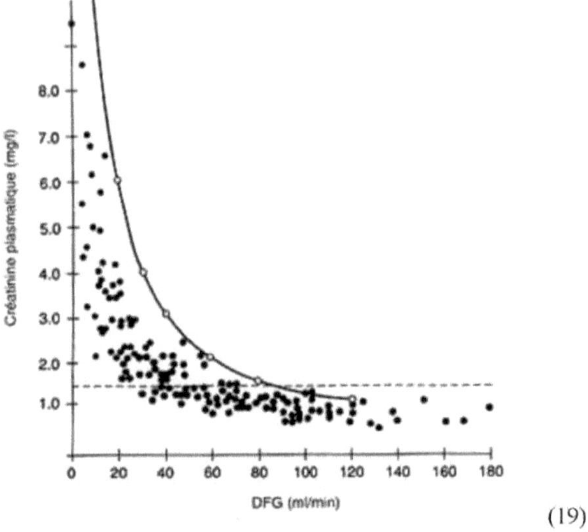

(19)

Figure 12: Relationship between glomerular filtration rate and creatinine levels.

The relationship between **glomerular filtration rate** and plasma creatinine level is non-linear, describing a hyperbolic curve (Fig.12).

This evidence is at the root of a first trap set for the clinician, who spontaneously tends to consider this relationship as linear, and thus to underestimate renal aggression.

3.4 Measuring creatinine clearance :

Creatinine clearance, defined as the amount of creatinine removed from plasma per unit time, is probably a more accurate indicator of glomerular filtration (20).

There are several formulas for calculating clearance from creatinine levels. However, it should be pointed out that various factors can influence its value.

- The Cockcroft and Gault formula thus integrates age, sex and weight:

$$clearance = \frac{(poids \times (140 - \hat{a}ge) \times 1{,}05\ (femme)\ ou\ 1{,}24\ (homme))}{cr\acute{e}atin\acute{e}mie}$$

- The MDRD (Modification of the Diet in Renal Disease) formula, subsequently developed, integrates age, sex, race, uremia and albuminemia:

$$170 \, x \, créatinémie^{-0.999} \, x \, age^{-0.176} \, x \, urée^{-0.170} \, x \, albuminémie^{+0.318} \, x \, (0,762 \text{ si femme})$$
$$\text{ou} \, x \, (1,18 \text{ si de race noire})$$

The clearances calculated from these formulas were consistent with each other and with inulin clearance for most patients (excluding those in intensive care).

The MDRD formula proved more reliable in patients over 65, and in obese patients.

These formulas do not take into account variations in urinary creatinine elimination or volume of distribution, which limits their use in resuscitation patients with acute renal failure (21).

In intensive care patients, the UV/P formula appears more reliable for assessing glomerular filtration rate.

Given the rapid variations in glomerular filtration rate in emergency and intensive care patients, we prefer to measure urinary creatinine on a sample collected over one hour and the mean of the creatinemia measured at the beginning and end of the interval. This measured creatinine clearance moderately overestimates glomerular filtration rate, due to tubular secretion of creatinine. Its values nevertheless remain well correlated.

Creatinine clearance therefore appears to be a good marker of glomerular filtration in intensive care patients, although threshold values have yet to be determined for defining and classifying renal aggression (22).

3.4 Cystatin C assay:

Cystatin C (formerly known as gamma-trace or post-gamma globulin) is a non-glycosylated, basic polypeptide (pH 9.3), composed of 122 amino acids and with a molecular weight of 13,359 daltons (23).

A member of the cysteine protease inhibitor family, this peptide protects against the destruction of cellular and extracellular tissues caused by the release of enzymes by dead or malignant cells.

Cystatin C is also thought to play a role in fighting infection. It is found in most body fluids, notably cerebrospinal fluid, where it was first identified and quantified.

Cystatin C is produced by all the nucleated cells studied.

There is no nycthemeral variation in blood levels of Cystatin C, and its production is not influenced by inflammation (24, 25).

The molecule's molecular weight and positive charge mean that it is freely filtered at the glomerular level. It is then almost entirely reabsorbed and catabolized in the proximal tubule.

Cystatin C concentration in urine is very low (except in cases of proximal tubulopathy).

The plasma concentration of Cystatin C therefore appears to be influenced only by glomerular filtration rate (26-28).

On the basis of clinical studies, we can conclude that serum Cystatin C concentration is a good marker of glomerular filtration rate compared with creatinine.

The sensitivity of Cystatin C may even be superior in certain well-defined patient subgroups. Its concentration is independent of muscle mass.

However, in view of the difference in price (the cost of Cystatin C is still much higher than that of creatinine). Further large-scale studies are still needed to confirm the value of this marker of glomerular filtration rate (29).

3.6 Other biological markers :

The literature evaluating the value of plasma or urine renal biomarkers is extremely rich (6).

Tubular biomarkers are indicators of renal tissue damage. The most widely studied are (30-32):

- Kidney Injury molecule-1 (KIM-1).
- Neutrophil gelatinase associated lipocalin (NGAL).
- Interleukin-18 (IL-18).
- β2-microglobulin.

These biomarkers primarily reflect the mechanism of renal aggression (ischemia, hypoxia, regeneration, etc.).

There are no real studies demonstrating their clinical usefulness in patients at risk of acute renal failure, and recommending their measurement for diagnostic purposes (33). They can be used to predict the onset of acute renal failure, to assess the risk of recourse to extra-renal purification and the risk of death in the intensive care setting (34) (Tab.1.2).

Table 1: Main biomarkers predictive of ARF in the ICU.

Marker	Sensitivity/specificity	sampling	Medium diagnosis
Gama GT and PAL	Sensitive non-specific	Urine	Auto-analyzer
NHE3	Specific	urine	Western blot
IL 18	Low-sensitivity specific		Elisa
NGAL	Early, sensitive and specific in urine.	Urine + blood	Elisa

(6)

Gamma GT: Gammglutamyl transferase; PAL: alkaline phosphatases; NHE3: H+/Na+ exchanger, IL18 interleukin 18, NGAL: neutrophil gelatinase-associated lipocalin.

Table 2: Predictive biomarkers for use of renal replacement therapy and death in the ICU.

Marker :	Sensitivity/specificity
IL 18	Not postponed
Cystatin C	Not postponed
NGAL	Sensitive and specific

(6)

3.5 Assessment of renal function using the U.V/ P formula:

The best practical assessment of glomerular filtration rate is made by the UV/P (ml/min) creatinine calculation formula.

U: urinary creatinine concentration in mmol/l
V: urine volume in ml related to time,
P: plasma creatinine concentration in mmol/l with urine collected for at least one hour.

If glomerular filtration rate (GFR) is to be measured, estimated formulas (Cockcroft-Gault, MDRD, CKD-EPI) should not be used in the intensive care or postoperative patient. The formula for calculating creatinine clearance (UV/P creatinine) should probably be used (33).

3.6 Assessment of renal function by hemodynamic methods :

Assessment of renal function by hemodynamic methods is based on evaluation of renal perfusion.

Three methods are used to assess renal perfusion:

- Contrast-enhanced ultrasound (CEUS)
- The semi-quantitative color Doppler renal perfusion assessment scale.
- Renal vascular resistance index.

3.8.1 Ultrasound with contrast :

Contrast-enhanced ultrasound (CEUS) (Fig.13) (35) is performed with a product consisting of microbubbles.

It is based on the use of microbubbles (composed of gas stabilized by a lipid or albumin envelope) injected into a peripheral vein.

These microbubbles are the same size as red blood cells and remain exclusively in the vascular space. As a result, they provide detailed images of tissue circulation.

After a bolus injection via a peripheral vein, assessment of the small circulation goes through several phases:

- An initial phase of cortical enhancement.

- A second phase of medullary contrast, starting in the outer medullary and

ending in the inner medullary.
* A third venous stage.

Microbubbles are inert and eliminated by the pulmonary route; they are not nephrotoxic, with rare anaphylactic reactions.

The European Society for Ultrasound in Medicine and Biology (EFSUMB) recommends other indications for contrast ultrasonography, namely (35):
* Diagnosis of renal parenchymal masses
* Investigation of renal vein thrombosis.
* Assessment of renal ischemic pathologies (renal infarction, cortical necrosis).

The use of contrast ultrasonography is recommended in patients with a contraindication to the use of iodinated contrast media or gadolinium salts.

The sensitivity of microbubbles to acoustic waves (microbubbles are destroyed under a high-frequency ultrasonographic beam) enables destruction-reperfusion sequences to be performed, providing a better approach to the quantitative study of renal perfusion (36).

Two indices are obtained by this technique and the ratio between these two indices reflects renal visceral perfusion:

* Average transit time.
* Relative blood volume.

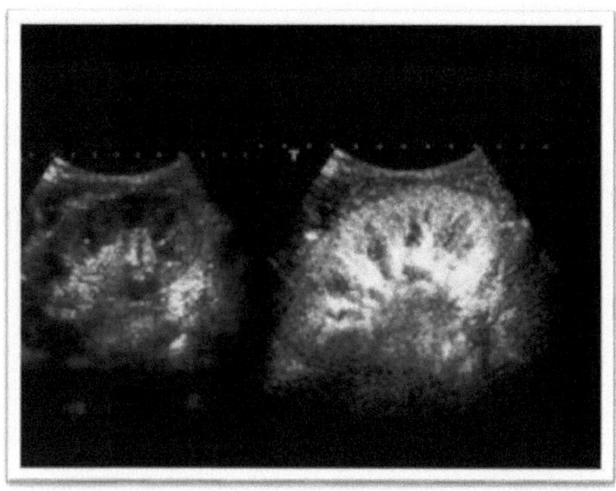

(36)

Figure 13: Ultrasound with contrast medium.
Human data highlight the heterogeneity of the results obtained and the lack of

correlation between indices derived from contrast-enhanced ultrasound and the various data on renal macro- and microcirculation.

3.8.2   Assessment of renal function by semi-quantitative color Doppler :

Exploration is generally performed with 2 to 5 MHZ probes, ideally convex, but an echocardiography probe may also be suitable (37, 38).

Obtaining a longitudinal section (Fig.14) of the kidney enables good visualization of vessels in color Doppler after reduction of the PRF (pulse repetition frequency), and quality measurements. A perfusion assessment scale has been proposed (39). (Tab.3).

Table 3: Semi-quantitative assessment of renal perfusion.

Grade	Renal perfusion assessed by color Doppler
0	No identifiable vessel
1	Some vessels visible in the hilum
2	Hilar and inter-lobar vessels visible in most parenchyma
3	Vessels visible up to the arcuate arteries in most of the parenchyma

This semi-quantitative assessment appears to be related to quantification by measurement of perfusion velocities (renal resistance index) (40, 41).

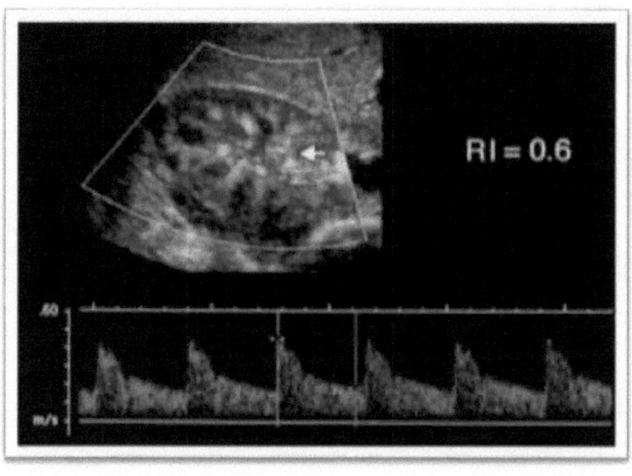

(41)

Figure 14: Semi-quantitative assessment combined with measurement of the renal resistance index.

3.8.3 Assessment of renal function by measuring the renal resistance index :

Non-invasive assessment of renal perfusion can be performed using renal Doppler ultrasound and measurement of the renal resistance index:

$$\textit{Index de résistance rénal } = \frac{\textit{Vitesse systolique} - \textit{Vitesse diastolique}}{\textit{Vitesse systolique}}$$

Assessment of renal perfusion by measuring the vascular resistance index offers several advantages over its evaluation by the semi-quantitative method or contrast ultrasonography (8) (Tab.4).

Table 4: Comparison of the three techniques used to assess renal perfusion.

	IRR	Semi-quantitative scale	Contrast ultrasonography
Benefits	Fast, non-invasive, reproducible and easy to learn.	Simple, reproducible, easy to learn	Perfusion-specific functional imaging
Disadvantages	Determines many measurement limit accuracies.	Subjective measurement	Specific equipment, cost, unproven reliability
Clinical applications	Renal prognosis	Renal prognosis	Optimizing renal hemodynamics
Level of evidence	Low to moderate	Low to moderate	Feasibility studies

(8)

Measurement of the renal resistance index ('RRI), which assesses renal perfusion using the Doppler method, appears to be straightforward, with a rapid learning curve and good inter-observer reproducibility (40).

This measurement can be carried out in the patient's bed, using probes with a frequency of 2 to 5 MHz. The posterior approach is often used, allowing visualization of the renal parenchyma (size, echostructure) (37, 38).

An initial semi-quantitative assessment of renal perfusion is performed by color Doppler while reducing PRF.

Pulsed Doppler analysis is continued after inter-lobar or arch arteries have been identified. The Doppler firing window is reduced to a minimum, and the spectrum is considered optimal when at least three successive cycles can be analyzed. Calculation of the renal resistance index, known as the Pourcelot index, is obtained by averaging measurements taken over three to five cycles. A value below 0.7 is considered normal.

Some authors have proposed the use of the pulsatility index as a method of assessing resistances (a method usually used for resistive profiles) (Fig.16).

The pulsatility index has been shown to correlate well with the renal resistance index (42). The only disadvantage of the pulsatility index is that it requires the measurement of mean velocity, and therefore of suitable software.

Limitations in interpreting renal resistance index values :

Clinical and experimental studies have shown little correlation between renal resistance index and renal vascular resistance and renal blood flow (42-44). The significance of the renal resistance index is therefore questionable.

In fact, this index essentially depends on two parameters:

- Vascular compliance (Fig.20): this explains the increase in the renal resistance index in certain pathologies such as arterial hypertension, diabetes and certain vasculitides, and its physiological increase with age (45-47).

-Transmural vascular pressure (TMP) (Fig.21): this represents a vascular distensibility pressure (intravascular pressure - extravascular pressure) which is reduced in the event of increased pressure in the renal parenchyma caused by interstitial edema in attacks and kidney damage (45, 46, 48).

This transmural pressure is increased in cases where there is an increase in locoregional blood flow.

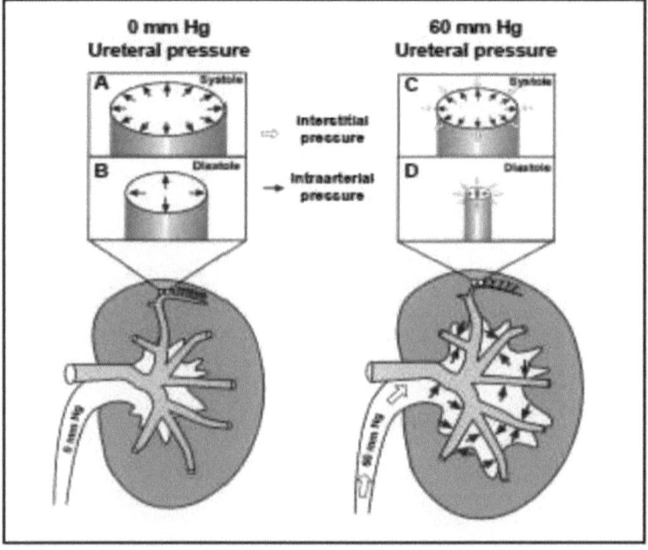

(41)

Figure 15: Impact of increased urinary tract pressure on parenchymal renal artery diameter.

Increased pressure in the renal parenchyma through increased pressure in the urinary tract influences systolo-diastolic flow in the distal renal arteries (41).

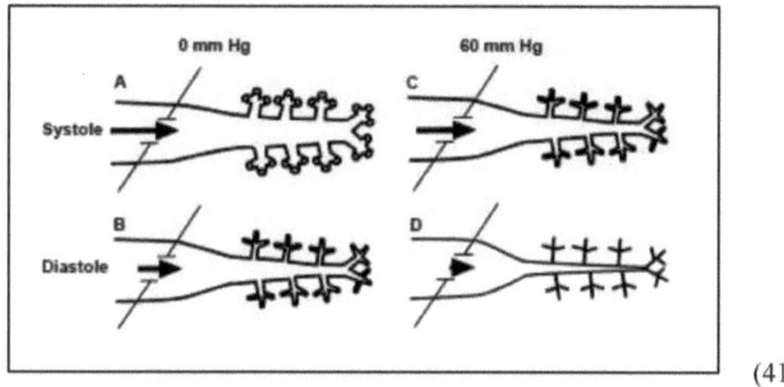

(41)

Figure 16: Impact of increased ureteral pressure on systolo-diastolic blood flow.

Various factors can influence the value of the renal resistance index (35):

- Age.
- Inhibitors of the renin-angiotensin-aldosterone system.
- Diabetic nephropathy.
- Renal artery stenoses (Fig. 16).
- Hypertensive nephropathies.
- Heart rate.
- Hydronephrosis (Fig. 17).
- Chronic kidney disease.
- Caffeine intake.
- A technical measurement error (insonation angle too open).

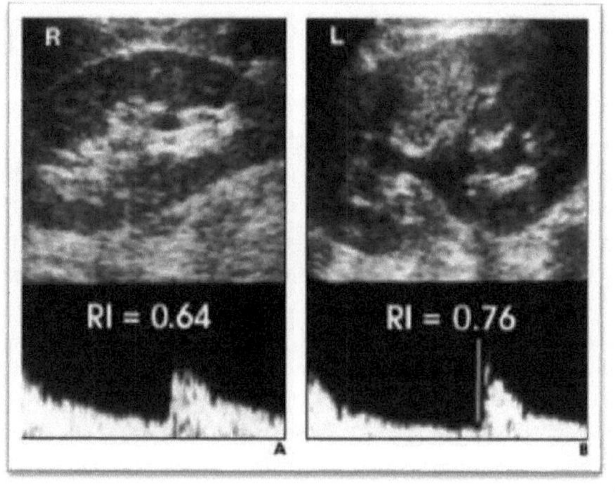

(41)

Figure 17: Impact of left ureteral obstruction on resistance index value.

Systolic and diastolic flow are greatly slowed in the event of renal artery obstruction (Fig.18) :

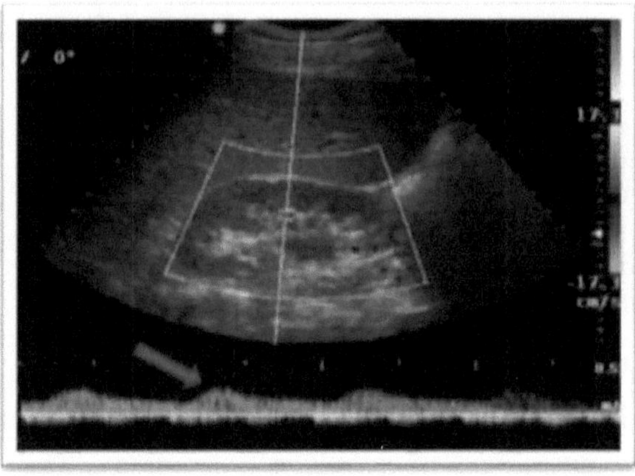

(51)

Figure 18: Impact of renal artery stenosis on parenchymal perfusion.

3.8.4   Renal resistance index in intensive care :

Several previous studies suggest a correlation between renal resistance index, renal vascular resistance and renal blood flow (49-52).

The renal resistance index has been used in intensive care to assess renal perfusion and the impact of certain therapies on renal perfusion, based on the principle that the prevention or treatment of renal damage depends first and foremost on improving renal perfusion:

This renal resistance index has been used in several practical applications:

- Early detection of kidney damage using a commonly used biological marker, creatininemia (12).
- Assessment of renal perfusion by administration of low doses of dopamine, and by a progressive change in mean arterial pressure level induced by a change in noradrenaline concentration (53).
- Early detection of occult hemorrhagic shock in polytrauma patients (54).
- Assessment of renal response to a filling test in intensive care patients (55, 56).
- Assessment of renal blood flow: in fact, there was no correlation between flow measured by Doppler-ultrasound and ultrasound transit time in the periphery, which is a validated method for measuring regional blood flow. Only variation in parenchymal diastolic velocity predicted a 20% variation in renal blood flow, but with an area under the ROC curve of moderate power (AUC-ROC = 0.75)(44).

- Prediction of acute renal failure :

In patients with septic shock, the index of resistance measured on admission was significantly higher in patients who developed acute renal failure in the days following admission. This index of resistance was also higher in a population of post-cardiac surgery patients requiring extracorporeal circulation (57).

- Differentiation between patients with persistent renal failure and those with reversible renal failure (12) (58, 59).

the resistance index probably has the same diagnostic performance for assessing short-term renal prognosis as the new plasma or urine biomarkers (60).

This index has also been used in a number of other clinical situations, as in :

- Management of general hemodynamics according to the value of the renal resistance index (filling, vasoactive amines) and assessment of urinary obstruction (61).
- Early detection of renal graft rejection (9).
- Prediction of the need for extra-renal purification (57).

Despite the practical interest of the question, the formalized expert recommendations (RFE 2015) does not support the use of this renal resistance index as a method of assessing renal function (62) :

> *« Il ne faut probablement pas utiliser l'index de résistance mesuré par le Doppler rénal pour diagnostiquer ou traiter une insuffisance rénale aiguë »*
>
> Recommandations grade 2 avec un accord fort.

The main limitations of this Doppler hemodynamic approach are the significance of variations in the renal resistance index, and the poor reproducibility of measurements. However, the potential clinical applications of this tool, the feasibility and reproducibility of the examination, and the absence of additional costs for a department already equipped with an ultrasound scanner, probably justify further investigations in this field.

4. Conclusion:

It must be emphasized that there is no relationship between renal perfusion, as assessed by the resistance index, and renal blood flow. The role of reduced RSF in the genesis of ischemic acute renal failure is now widely questioned. Pre-conditioning phenomena appearing in response to a few hours' exposure to hypoxia have been reported to protect against the secondary onset of renal injury. The aim of lowering RDS is to reduce sodium intake and active sodium reabsorption, thereby reducing O2 consumption.

Some studies have found that the renal resistance index has acceptable validity for diagnosing and predicting the risk of acute renal failure. Assessing the severity and reversibility of renal damage using the same index has proved to be an interesting diagnostic tool.

The study of renal perfusion by measuring the renal resistance index shows statistically significant relationships with many parameters (age, body mass index, heart rate, etc.). The most interesting correlations were found with the gold standard used to diagnose acute renal failure, represented by diuresis and creatininemia. This index of vascular resistance also influenced the overall evolution of patients (deaths, discharges and transfers) [63].

Widely accepted as factors influencing organ perfusion, parameters of general hemodynamics (mean arterial pressure, systolo-diastolic pressures, blood volume and ventricular function) do not necessarily influence the quality of renal perfusion, as assessed by measurement of the renal resistance index.

In the other results observed, we noted the absence of correlations between the value of the renal resistance index and the concentrations of various sympathomimetic drugs (Dobutamine, adrenaline, noradrenaline) which is also observed in the various data in the literature despite the use of different vasopressor agents. [63]

Assessment of renal perfusion using the Doppler method seems to be an easy-to-learn, easy-to-perform, non-invasive and harmless-to-repeat diagnostic tool, which above all makes it possible to identify patients at risk of renal damage, and to predict the severity and evolution of this damage after diagnostic confirmation using conventional criteria (creatinemia and diuresis).

In our department, the principle of using a single ultrasound probe (the cardiac probe) to perform the maximum number of radiological explorations, starting with the heart and thorax, and passing through the brain and abdomen as part of the protocol for exploring the various medical distresses (neurological, hemodynamic and respiratory), the rapid exploration of the renal parenchyma and its vascularization using the Doppler method does not appear to significantly prolong the time required for the overall ultrasound examination, compared with the information that can be provided in search of renal damage, which on its own and independently represents a non-negligible factor in morbidity and mortality.

This notion of assessing renal perfusion in situations at risk of renal failure must be taken into account in the perioperative and trauma settings as part of the ultrasound FAST protocol.

The use of the resistance index to assess renal perfusion as a method of diagnosing renal failure has so far failed to replace conventional diagnostic criteria (KDIGO). The only performance of this index found in the various studies lies in the prediction of the risk of renal damage, which could make it possible to optimize the means of renal protection in the medical and surgical environment, starting with the re-establishment of an effective blood volume, an acceptable mean perfusion pressure, and ending with the non-aggravation of renal lesions by limiting the use of potentially nephrotoxic products.

The use of this technique to assess renal perfusion should in no way replace the basic management and monitoring of renal function, i.e. quantification of diuresis and plasma measurement of the classic marker, creatinine.

What we can recommend is that the non-invasive study of renal perfusion by Doppler should be used in all patients at risk of acute renal failure. Even in the absence of KDIGO diagnostic criteria, this investigation will make it possible to anticipate the various therapeutic measures aimed at preventing, limiting and not aggravating acute renal injury. [63]

Once renal damage has been confirmed by conventional clinical-biological criteria (creatininemia and diuresis), the use of Doppler measurement will enable us, in addition to hemodynamic measures to improve renal parenchymal perfusion, to assess the severity and predict the course of this acute renal failure.

The limitations observed in the use of creatinine for the diagnosis of acute renal failure are the basis for the development of new markers of renal impairment. Many markers have been evaluated for different purposes, namely the diagnostic prediction of acute renal failure, and the assessment of the severity and prognosis of this renal damage. The ideal marker should be simple, non-invasive and have a good sensitivity/specificity ratio with good reproducibility.

Assessment of renal perfusion by Doppler measurement of the vascular resistance index, or by other methods, appears to be a powerful tool with promising diagnostic power in the global evaluation of renal function.

For the time being, it is not recommended to use renal perfusion as a diagnostic tool for acute renal failure, since the gold standard for diagnosing AKI remains the combination of the two clinico-biological criteria, i.e. creatininemia and diuresis.

BIBLIOGRAPHY :

1.   Ostermann M, Chang RW. Acute kidney injury in the intensive care unit according to RIFLE. Critical care medicine. 2007;35(8):1837-43.
2.   Hoste EA, Schurgers M. Epidemiology of acute kidney injury: how big is the problem? Critical care medicine. 2008;36(4):S146-S51.
3.   Bagshaw SM. Short-and long-term survival after acute kidney injury. Oxford University Press; 2008.
4.   Bagshaw SM, George C, Dinu I, Bellomo R. A multi-centre evaluation of the RIFLE criteria for early acute kidney injury in critically ill patients. Nephrology Dialysis Transplantation. 2007;23(4):1203-10.
5.   Le Gall C, Jacob L. Insufflsance rénale alguë en réanImatlon: quels crltères? quelle classIflcatIon? Mapar; 2011.
6.   Du Cheyron D, Terzi N, Charbonneau P. New biological markers of acute renal failure. Réanimation. 2008;17(8):775-82.
7.   Lerolle N. Use of the renal vascular resistance index measured by Doppler ultrasound during septic shock. Réanimation. 2009;18(8):708-13.
8.   Schnell D, Darmon M. What is the place of renal Doppler in the management of acute renal failure? Intensive Care Medicine. 2016;25(6):570-7.
9.   Radermacher J, Mengel M, Ellis S, Stuht S, Hiss M, Schwarz A, et al. The renal arterial resistance index and renal allograft survival. New England Journal of Medicine. 2003;349(2):115-24.
10.   Mostbeck GH, Zontsich T, Turetschek K. Ultrasound of the kidney: obstruction and medical diseases. European radiology. 2001;11(10):1878-89.
11.   Audren N. Are renal vascular resistance index and Neutrophil Gelatinase Associated Lipocalin assay markers of acute renal failure after cardiac surgery? 2012.
12.   Darmon M, Schortgen F, Vargas F, Liazydi A, Schlemmer B, Brun-Buisson C, et al. Diagnostic accuracy of Doppler renal resistive index for reversibility of acute kidney injury in critically ill patients. Intensive care medicine. 2011;37(1):68-76.
13.   Godin-Ribuot D. Renal physiologies The nephron and renal circulation. ECN.(Université Joseph Fourier - Grenoble 1) ed. Grenoble: (Université Joseph Fourier - Grenoble 1); 2011/2012.
14.   Ader Jl. Renal physiology. ECN, editor. Paris: MASSON; 2013 2016. 664 p.
15.   Kerbi. renal physiology; Academic year 2015-2016; Université Badji Mokhtar Annaba. université Badji Mokhtar Annaba2015/2016.
16.   Gueutin V. Le Manuel Du Résident Néphrologie 2017. 2017 ed. 75013 Paris, France2017 300 p.
17.   Bensouna. Physiological role of the Renal Circulation and Regulation of Glomerular Filtration. Faculty of Medicine: OUARGLA; Academic year 2018/2019.
18.   Dieusaert P, Deweerdt L. Guide pratique des analyses médicales. Lyon Pharmaceutique. 1996;5(47):271.
19.   Shemesh O, Golbetz H, KRIss JP, Myers BD. Limitations of creatinine as a filtration marker in glomerulopathic patients. Kidney international. 1985;28(5):830-8.
20.   Cockcroft DW, Gault MH. Prediction of Creatinine Clearance from Serum Creatinine°. Nephron. 1976;16:31-41.
21.   Poggio ED, Wang X, Greene T, Van Lente F, Hall PM. Performance of the modification of diet in renal disease and Cockcroft-Gault equations in the estimation of GFR in health and in chronic kidney disease. Journal of the American Society of

Nephrology. 2005;16(2):459-66.

22.   Novis BK, Roizen MF, Aronson S, Thisted RA. Association of preoperative risk factors with postoperative acute renal failure. Anesthesia and analgesia. 1994;78(1):143-9.

23.   CH R. Diagnostic applications of cystatin C. In: 2000 BJBS, editor. Diagnostic applications of cystatin C: biomed; 2000.

24.   Cimerman N, Brguljan PM, Krasovec M, Suskovic S, Kos J. Twenty-four hour variations of cystatin C and total cysteine proteinase inhibitory activity in sera from healthy subjects. Clinica chimica acta. 2000;1(291):89-95.

25.   Randers E, Kornerup K, Erlandsen EJ, Hasling C, Danielsen H. Cystatin C levels in sera of patients with acute infectious diseases with high C-reactive protein levels. Scandinavian journal of clinical and laboratory investigation. 2001;61(4):333-5.

26.   Lofberg H, Grubb A. Quantitation of y-trace in human biological fluids: indications for production in the central nervous system. Scandinavian journal of clinical and laboratory investigation.
1979;39(7):619-26.

27.   Grubb A. Diagnostic value of analysis of cystatin C and protein HC in biological fluids. Clinical nephrology. 1992;38:S20-7.

28.   Uchida K, Gotoh A. Measurement of cystatin-C and creatinine in urine. Clinica chimica acta. 2002;323(1-2):121-8.

29.   Delanaye P, Chapelle J-P, Gielen J, Krzesinski J-M, Rorive G. The value of cystatin C in the evaluation of renal function. Nephrology. 2003;24(8):457-68.

30.   Kdigo A. Work Group. KDIGO clinical practice guideline for acute kidney injury. Kidney Int Suppl. 2012;2(1):1-138.

31.   Cruz DN, Mehta RL. Acute kidney injury in 2013: Breaking barriers for biomarkers in AKI-- progress at last. Nature reviews Nephrology. 2014;10(2):74.

32.   Parikh CR1 DP. New biomarkers of acute kidney injury.

33.   Réanimation GF, Pédiatriques U, Ichai C, Vinsonneau C, Souweine B, Canet E, et al. ACUTE RENAL INSUFFICIENCY IN PERIOPERATIVE AND RESUSCITATION (Excluding extrarenal purification techniques) RFE commune SFAR-SRLF.

34.   Ahlstrom A, Tallgren M, Peltonen S, Pettila V. Evolution and predictive power of serum cystatin C in acute renal failure. Clinical nephrology. 2004;62(5):344-50.

35.   Pruijm M, Ponte B, Hofmann L, Vogt B, Eisenberger U, Meuwly J, et al. New radiological techniques to investigate patients suffering from chronic kidney disease. Revue medicale suisse. 2011;7(284):505-9.

36.   Le Dorze M, Bouglé A, Deruddre S, Duranteau J. Renal Doppler ultrasound: a new tool to assess renal perfusion in critical illness. Shock. 2012;37(4):360-5.

37.   Schnell D, Darmon M. Renal Doppler to assess renal perfusion in the critically ill: a reappraisal. Intensive care medicine. 2012;38(11):1751-60.

38.   Schnell D, Darmon M. Bedside Doppler ultrasound for the assessment of renal perfusion in the ICU: advantages and limitations of the available techniques. Springer; 2015.

39.   Barozzi L, Valentino M, Santoro A, Mancini E, Pavlica P. Renal ultrasonography in critically ill patients. Critical care medicine. 2007;35(5):S198-S205.

40.   Schnell D, Reynaud M, Venot M, Le AM, Dinic M, Baulieu M, et al. Resistive Index or color- Doppler semi-quantitative evaluation of renal perfusion by inexperienced physicians: results of a pilot study. Minerva anestesiologica. 2014;80(12):1273-81.

41.   Tublin ME, Bude RO, Platt JF. The resistive index in renal Doppler sonography:

where do we stand? American Journal of Roentgenology. 2003;180(4):885-92.

42.   Bude RO, Rubin JM. Relationship between the resistive index and vascular compliance and resistance. Radiology. 1999;211(2):411-7.

43.   Murphy ME, Tublin ME. Understanding the Doppler RI: impact of renal arterial distensibility on the RI in a hydronephrotic ex vivo rabbit kidney model. Journal of ultrasound in medicine. 2000;19(5):303-14.

44.   Wan L, Yang N, Hiew C-Y, Schelleman A, Johnson L, May C, et al. An assessment of the accuracy of renal blood flow estimation by Doppler ultrasound. Intensive care medicine. 2008;34(8):1503-10.

45.   Derchi LE, Leoncini G, Parodi D, Viazzi F, Martinoli C, Ratto E, et al. Mild renal dysfunction and renal vascular resistance in primary hypertension. American journal of hypertension. 2005;18(7):966-71.

46.   Ohta Y, Fujii K, Arima H, Matsumura K, Tsuchihashi T, Tokumoto M, et al. Increased renal resistive index in atherosclerosis and diabetic nephropathy assessed by Doppler sonography. Journal of hypertension. 2005;23(10):1905-11.

47.   Terry JD, Rysavy JA, Frick MP. Intrarenal Doppler: characteristics of aging kidneys. Journal of Ultrasound in Medicine. 1992;11(12):647-51.

48.   Mitchell GF. Effects of central arterial aging on the structure and function of the peripheral vasculature: implications for end-organ damage. Journal of applied physiology. 2008;105(5):1652-60.

49.   Tublin ME, Tessler FN, Murphy ME. Correlation between renal vascular resistance, pulse pressure, and the resistive index in isolated perfused rabbit kidneys. Radiology. 1999;213(1):258-64.

50.   Duranteau J, Deruddre S, Vigue B, Chemla D. Doppler monitoring of renal hemodynamics: why the best is yet to come. Springer; 2008.

51.   Granata A, Zanoli L, Clementi S, Fatuzzo P, Di Nicolò P, Fiorini F. Resistive intrarenal index: myth or reality? The British journal of radiology. 2014;87(1038):20140004.

52.   Mostbeck G, Gossinger H, Mallek R, Siostrzonek P, Schneider B, Tscholakoff D. Effect of heart rate on Doppler measurements of resistive index in renal arteries. Radiology. 1990;175(2):511-3.

53.   Lauschke A, Teichgraber U, Frei U, Eckardt K-U. Low-dose dopamine worsens renal perfusion in patients with acute renal failure. Kidney international. 2006;69(9):1669-74.

54.   Corradi F, Brusasco C, Vezzani A, Palermo S, Altomonte F, Moscatelli P, et al. Hemorrhagic shock in polytrauma patients: early detection with renal Doppler resistive index measurements. Radiology. 2011;260(1):112-8.

55.   Schnell D, Camous L, Guyomarc'h S, Duranteau J, Canet E, Gery P, et al. Renal perfusion assessment by renal Doppler during fluid challenge in sepsis. Critical care medicine. 2013;41(5):1214-20.

56.   Moussa MD, Scolletta S, Fagnoul D, Pasquier P, Brasseur A, Taccone FS, et al. Effects of fluid administration on renal perfusion in critically ill patients. Critical care. 2015;19(1):250.

57.   Bossard G, Bourgoin P, Corbeau J, Huntzinger J, Beydon L. Early detection of postoperative acute kidney injury by Doppler renal resistive index in cardiac surgery with cardiopulmonary bypass. British journal of anaesthesia. 2011;107(6):891-8.

58.   Schnell D, Deruddre S, Harrois A, Pottecher J, Cosson C, Adoui N, et al. Renal resistive index better predicts the occurrence of acute kidney injury than cystatin C. Shock. 2012;38(6):592-7.

59.   Izumi M, Sugiura T, Nakamura H, Nagatoya K, Imai E, Hori M. Differential diagnosis of prerenal azotemia from acute tubular necrosis and prediction of recovery by Doppler ultrasound. American journal of kidney diseases. 2000;35(4):713-9.

60.   Dewitte A, Joannes-Boyau O, Sidobre C, Fleureau C, Bats M-L, Derache P, et al. Kinetic eGFR and novel AKI biomarkers to predict renal recovery. Clinical Journal of the American Society of Nephrology. 2015;10(11):1900-10.

61.   Deruddre S, Cheisson G, Mazoit J-X, Vicaut E, Benhamou D, Duranteau J. Renal arterial resistance in septic shock: effects of increasing mean arterial pressure with norepinephrine on the renal resistive index assessed with Doppler ultrasonography. Intensive care medicine. 2007;33(9):1557-62.

62.   Ichai C, Vinsonneau C, Souweine B, Canet E, Clec'h C, Constantin J-M, et al. Acute renal failure in perioperative and intensive care (excluding extrarenal purification techniques). Intensive care medicine. 2017;26(6):481-504.

63.   L.ghanem lakhal. Index de résistance rénal et évaluation de l'hémodynamique intra-rénale dans les insuffisances circulatoires.thèse de doctorat en sciences médicales 2020. Constantine 3 University

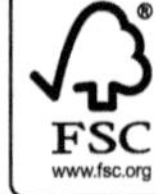